Also by Dr. Stenbeck

Available from the usual on-line source

Books

Healing Yourself -- The Holistic Approach
   [An introduction to Holistic Self-healing.]

Heal Yourself Right Now!
   [The Seven Priority Organ Levels for
   effective Nutritional/Holistic Treatment of
   all organs.]

The 22 Unique Body Types
   (for Health and Weight Loss)

Q & A to Identify Your Body Type (Booklet)
   [Individual Type booklets are available]

Booklets
(Step-by-step instructions on healing yourself)

   #1 Start Healing with Positive Thinking
   #2 Mastering Positive Feelings for Health!
   #3 Spiritual Balance and Your Healing

The Nervimotive Body Type

The Frank Sinatra, Elizabeth Taylor Celebrity Body Type

For Kaye,
there at the beginning with Doc Severn,
and for Liberty,
continuing the holistic healing journey…

Disclaimer

The information in this book is for educational purposes only and is not a substitute for medication, diets, or other medical care. The diets do not treat diseases or medical conditions, and are an adjunct to your orthodox health care.

The author and publisher accept no responsibility for any misuse of the information within. If you have any physical problem, food allergy, emotional disorder, or disease, common sense dictates that you consult with a physician before changing your diet, taking nutritional supplements, or following the advice given here.

About the Author

Educated in New Zealand and in the U.S.A., Dr. Stenbeck attained B.Sc. (NZ), M.S., and D.C. degrees. His holistic healing methods have been profiled in magazines (Esquire, McLean's, Playgirl, the Atlanta Constitution), and on TV in the USA and in Canada. He was the main contributor to the Warner Book, _The Eye/Body Connection_ by Jessica Maxwell that focused on the holistic healing relationships between the iris structure and organ genetics.

In the 1970-80's he was elected Fellow, Royal Society of Health, London; Fellow, American Association of Chemists; Member, American Association of Clinical Chemists; and Affiliate, Royal Society of Medicine, London. He studied naturopathy and Body Types with Dr. Bernard Jensen and Dr. Clifford Severn, and has practiced in medical partnerships where patients received the joint benefits of medical and holistic healing.

He is a member of Self-Realization Fellowship. To receive advice on any health issue from a holistic viewpoint, or to receive help with your body type, see his web site: *DrStenbeck.net*

———

Contents

* * *

The Nervimotive Body Type (and Food Guide)   *1*

Appendix

* * *

The 22 Body Types:
Celebrity Examples

This Booklet contains the **Nervimotive** *type.
[See* <u>*The 22 Unique Body Types*</u> *for all type descriptions.]*

Thin Types

Atrophic   Woody Allen / Audrey Hepburn
Stan Laurel / Calista Flockheart

Exesthesic   Cher / Sarah Jessica Parker
(Female type only)

Marasmic   President Obama / Princess Diana
James Stewart / Kate Blanchard

Neurogenic   J.K. Simmons / Joan Rivers
Jon Cryer / Marin Hinle

Pathoferic   (No celebrity males)
Blythe Danner / Gwyneth Paltrow

Sillevitic   David Bowie / Shirley MacLaine
Rod Stewart / Carol Channing

Muscle Types

Calciferic	*Michael Jordan / Angelica Huston* *Abraham Lincoln / Grace Jones*
Carbogenic	*George Clooney / Lady Gaga* *Pres. G. Bush, Jr. / Meg Ryan*
Desmogenic	*Marlon Brando / Loni Anderson* *Daniel Craig / Tina Turner*
Eldic	*Ross Perot / Hillary Clinton* *Peter Falk / Sigourney Weaver*
Myogenic	*Pres. Bill Clinton / Sharon Stone* *Pres. John Kennedy / Julia Roberts*
Nervimotive	*Frank Sinatra / Elizabeth Taylor* *Mark Wahlberg / Natalie Wood*
Nitropheric	*Ben Affleck / Ava Gardner* *Kirk Douglas / Kate Winslet*
Pallinomic	*Pres. Donald Trump /* *Attorney General Janet Reno* *Bill O'Reilly (Fox) / Jane Russell*

Fat Types

Barotic
Robin Williams / "Mrs. Doubtfire"
Elton John / William Conrad

Carboferic
Bill Murray / Roseanne
Billy Gardell / Melissa McCarthy

Hydripheric
John Goodman / Shelly Winters
Wayne Knight / Jennifer Holliday

Isogenic
Einstein / Oprah Winfrey
Phillip S. Hoffman / Queen Victoria

Lipopheric
Rush Limbaugh / Rosie O'Donnell
Chris Christie / Camryn Manheim

Oxypheric
Winston Churchill / Orsen Welles
Ella Fitzgerald / Gerry Spence

Pargenic
Burt Reynolds / Katey Segal
Ron Perlman / Kirstey Alley

Succinct Quote on Human Types

From Victor Rocine, who first described discrete body types around 1900.

"A type is an order of people that differentiates and distinguishes itself by a general and similar form, brain-formation, chemistry, structure, build, immunity, tendencies, predisposition, resemblance, skin-pigment, and type characteristics based on observation and analogy.

"Or, in other words, people of a given type are similar physically and like-minded as if they were brothers and sisters—that is what type means.

"Everything in nature is made according to plan. Man only discovers that plan and gives it a name. The zoologist has not made the animals—he has only described the plan adopted by the wonderful Creator, and named the classes, subclasses, etc.

"How important type research will be to humanity, time alone will make known."

———

Prologue

The esteemed scientist J. J. Berzelius, discoverer of several chemical elements, inspired Victor Rocine to research body types and to investigate the correlation between types and their diseases. Around 1890-1910, Rocine privately published his original findings on the mineral basis of different body types, and this present book exists because of his brilliant insights.

For many years, I studied with Dr. Clifford Severn who had been a personal student of Victor Rocine on body types, naturopathy, herbology, iris analysis, diet, and nutritional healing methods. He had a successful career as a lecturer and healer, and was one of those rare athletes with complete muscle control over his body. I saw him under a spotlight at 85 years of age, contracting and rippling every individual muscle in his perfectly developed body. Field-Marshal Jan Smuts, the WWII South African Prime Minister, devoted a full chapter of his autobiography to how Severn's healing methods had saved his life. In the 1950's, *Life* magazine did a four-page spread on Severn and his family. Fame he had.

Another Rocine student I studied with, Dr. Bernard Jensen wrote of Rocine's body type research and nutritional methods in his privately published book *The Chemistry of Man*.

This book is deeply rooted in Rocine's original work, and with that of Herbert Shelton, M.D., Ph.D. (at Harvard University in the 1930's). I integrated their research with newer dietary and nervous system data along with celebrity examples of each type, hopefully, making this material easier to digest and more entertaining for the reader.

Gayelord Hauser, another Rocine student I knew, was a celebrated health book author. He wrote a popular book on Rocine's types in the 1940's, *Types and Temperaments;* reputedly, he also introduced yogurt to the western world.

This book exists because of Rocine's creative brilliance and original discoveries in natural healing.

▶ *Rocine: "The soul creates the body type."*

Rocine taught that the soul chooses a body type and brain to live in, thus presenting different experiences and life lessons to master. Why were *you* born the way you are?

That is something to think about, especially if it is true! What would your soul purpose be to live in a particular body type. I provide some thoughts on this issue in each type description and try to assess from my experience with your type the particular lessons of life presented therein.

Rocine was as brilliant in his way as an Abraham Lincoln, Michael Jordan, Michael Phelps, Tony Robbins, or a Daniel Day Lewis—all *calciferics*—rare, leaders, innovative, brilliant, and highly intelligent in their different fields of endeavor.

Celebrity examples exist for most types, not a duplicate of you, but someone who has your essence in their body-mind individuality. Knowing your type allows you to become a better you!

The celebrity examples provide further help in identifying your body type.

▶ *Rocine's classic findings are the backbone of this book. Integrated with Sheldon's research and with other dietary and food issues including mental, emotional, and spiritual attributes,*

Many people take nutritional supplements and try different diets without a doctor's advice. If this is your choice, use common sense, listen to body responses, and discontinue any allergic reactions to foods or nutritional substances.

———

The Nervimotive Body Type

Representing one of the 22 Body Types first described by Victor Rocine around 1900

***

"*You may also have a physical or psychological feature not representative of your type such as height, weight, appearance, talent, weakness, strength, etc., due to biochemical errors, environmental influences, racial or cultural differences, and congenital or genetic issues. Nevertheless, the type identification of the average persons is usually clear.*"

— *Victor Rocine*

Nervimotive Type Celebrity Examples

*If you think this is your type, be sure to look at **on-line photographs** of these examples. Look for general similarities to yourself. Note that sub-types cause the differences in appearance between members of the same type.*

ROYALTY

Queen Elizabeth II

ACTORS (many Oscars!)

Frank Sinatra	Matt Dillon
Mark Wahlberg	Eddie Murphy
Tim Allen	Jack Lemon
Bob Hope	Sean Penn
Tom Skerrit	Al Pacino
Charlie Chaplin	Errol Flynn
Roy Scheider	Steve McQueen
Douglas Fairbanks, Jr.	Brad Davis
Henry Winkler	Ronald Coleman
Everett Sloane	Paul Hogan
George Chakaris	Don Hamm
Robert Wagner	

Selma Heyak   Penelope Cruz
Jennifer Tilly   Bette Davis
Elizabeth Taylor   Natalie Wood
Sandra Bullock   Susan Sarandon
Julia Louis-Dreyfus   Karen Allen
Marie Tomei   Lesley Ann
Mary Elizabeth Mastrantonio

TV

Dennis Miller   Johnny Carson
Geraldo Rivera   Arsenio Hall
Paul Reiser   Michael J. Fox
Rami Malek ("Mr. Robot")
Marina Sirtis Troy   Fran Drescher

VOICE

John Lennon   Bobby Darin
Sammy Davis Jr.
Gloria Estefan   Prince

SPORTS

Joe Namath   Joe Montana
Sugar Ray Leonard   Michael Chang
Jimmy Connors   Rafeal Nadal
John McEnroe (many tennis players and
boxers)
Mark Spitz (multiple U.S.A. Olympic Golds)
Florence Griffin-Joyner (Olympic)

ARTS/OTHER

Ralph Nader	Ringo Starr
Carlos Castenada	
Heidi Fleiss	Gloria Allred

[Note: I knew three of the above celebrities, many others in everyday life and in my family, which contributed to my understanding of the type.

You already know something about this type from their public persona and appearance, whether from seeing them yourself or from the celebrity examples. Blend such insights with the type descriptions and the types of your family and friends to discern their presence in your midst!

Read the types, and if still confused you may choose to use the personal request for type identification from the web site: *DrStenbeck.net*

———

Nervimotive Type Questionnaire

Other than for the physical descriptions, these questions describe the generic type, and not specifically you! If any question ever applied to you, then choose he True answer!

For Question 1 only
  A = True   *B = Maybe*   *C = Untrue*
15 points   *7 points*   *1 point*

1. Physically identify with celebrity example____

Then...

  A = True   *B = Maybe*   *C = Untrue*
15 points   *3 points*   *1 point*

---

2. Height is close to:
   Males: 5'0-6'1   Females: 4'9-5'8   ____
3. Usual weight is close to:
   Males: 130-220 Females: 90-160   ____
4. Body slender or medium-sized; weight relatively easily controlled (unless have a fat sub-type)   ____
5. Compact moderately strong muscles   ____
6. Have a nervous nature; easily stressed   ____
7. Give 110% until drop from exhaustion ____
8. Attracted to power, education, reputation, position   ____

9. Square-rectangular forehead; on profile may have a vertical forehead ____

10. Mouth may be terse; upper lip often thin; lower lip variable in shape ____

11. Face is large at cheekbones; bony face; vertical lines in cheeks common ____

12. Wide lower jaw angles; jaw usually slopes as a straight line to the chin ____

13. Have good business judgment ____

14. Nose usually small, snub; some large ____

15. Lungs large and strong; male chest often hairy; medium or large bust ____

16. Highly impassioned ____

17. Strongly idealist, will fight for a cause ____

18. Excellent ability to socialize and converse with people ____

19. Hair lovely, dark, brunette; often grays in 20-30's ____

20. Hairline straight across forehead; "widow peak" common ____

22. High executive and management skills ____

23. Good sense of humor ____

24. Desire obedience from others ____

25. May be aggressive and pushy ____

26. Easily become impatient or excitable ____

27. Impulsive; will act on a dare ____

28. Believe in an "eye for an eye" ____

29. Readily pursue law suits ____

30. Tend to "know-it-all" based on certainty you are right; want others to accept your views ____

31. Very expressive with feelings ____

32. Have high self-confidence _____
33. Are goal-oriented _____
34. May have awkward jerky movements of some part of body (males mostly) _____
35. Talents in talking, teaching, legal, acting, literary, finances, intellectual _____
36. Are not diplomats or scientists _____
37. Are carnivorous (enjoy flesh); few ever become vegetarian _____
38. Have bravado, boasting, cockiness _____
39. Voice is cool and matter-of-fact _____
40. High endurance and adrenaline _____
41. Fussy, proud and impatient _____
42. Moderate to strong sexual drive _____
43. Powerful and active willpower _____
44. Brave and responsive in emergencies _____
45. Mentally strong _____
46. Seek retribution fro hurts and slights _____
47. Feel deeply, express feelings as felt _____
48. History of digestive problems _____
49. Have difficulty handling stress of life _____
50. Very social: able to talk for hours _____
51. Industrious, practical, hard-working _____
52. Gifted, artistic, sensitive _____
53. Easily irritated; bad temper in some _____
54. Often brilliant _____
55. May be mystical and intuitive _____
56. Take bold and immediate action _____
57. Voice can be loud and passionate (or controlled) _____
58. Manners are coarse and perfunctory _____
59. Are impatient and demanding _____

60. Genetics and diet are carnivorous   ____
61. Back, shoulders broad, square,
    strong and muscular   ____
62. Highly motivated   ____
63. Have great judgment in business   ____
64. Are intense, easily irritated   ____
65. Often impatient, excitable, intolerant   ____
66. Often impulsive and unpredictable   ____

Scoring

For question #1:
    A response: give 15 points   =_____
    B response: give 7 points   =_____
    C response: give 1 points   =_____

For questions #2—66:
    A response: give 5 points   =_____
    B response: give 3 points   =_____
    C response: give 1 point   =_____

Total of the above points   =_____

Interpretation
166—310: PROBABLY Nervimotive
90—165: POSSIBLY Nervimotive type
   <90: NOT Nervimotive type

The Nervimotive Type

Rocine: "Nervi-motive means 'motivated by nervous intensity.'" You utilize more <u>calcium, phosphorus, and sulfur</u> than other types, and easily become phosphorus deficient.

———

Your nervous system is truly on a go-go schedule! Your body type is a combination of strong muscle, nerve, and bone systems. The females are usually of short to medium-height (often less than five feet in Latin and oriental countries). The men come in all heights, some at six feet. You have a strong, angular body with longer limbs and a shorter trunk; your movements may be awkward. Many Oriental, Latin, Spanish, and Middle-Eastern people are of your type. Mark Spitz, the USA Olympic multiple Gold Medalist swimmer, personifies the physical perfection and performance your type may achieve (with a muscular sub-type). Sugar Ray Leonard and many excellent boxers are also your type.

You vary considerably in appearance, from being plain-looking to the ruggedly handsome men (Steve McQueen, Frank Sinatra, Johnny Carson, Errol Flynn), to the beautiful and exquisite ladies (Selma Heyak, Pentelope Cruz, Elizabeth Taylor, Natalie Wood, Lesley Ann Warren. Marcia Clark.

―――

Physical Similarity to Other Types

The *neurogenic* type (President Eisenhower, Jane Seymour) has a similar build, but when the *nervimotive* moves and talks, the differences are clear especially in the females (see the following comparison chart).

The *eldic* type (Ross Perot, Shirley MacLaine) is ethical, and controlling.

The *medeic* type (David Caruso, Madonna) is lean, and less congenial.

―――

Average Height and Weight

Males:	5'0-6'1	130-220 pounds
Females:	4'9-5'8	90-160 pounds

―――

Nervimotive Type Description

The type description represents how you appear in everyday society. You may have a sub-type that alters parts of this description.

Think of the celebrity examples as you read the descriptions. You are born to be slender, but with a fatty sub-type, there may be a life-long fight with weight (Elizabeth Taylor). Your medium-sized muscular body is usually of moderate strength. Your body comes with many looks, sizes, and shapes, and identifying your body takes practice. You are most often confused with *neurogenics* (which often is your sub-type, moderating your personality traits).

▶ *Rocine: "There are many variations in your head features, perhaps more-so than in any other type."*

Head —Your head comes in many variations, some are wedge-shaped, large above and behind the ears; others have a flat, small back-head, and are wide between the ears. Your forehead is square and wide from side to side, and it may be vertical on a profile view.

Hair —Your hairline is often straight across the forehead with a widow's peak being common (as in many females). If healthy, your hair is thick and lovely; nervous intensity causes your dark and stiff hair to gray early. The males look good with a moustache. You maintain a full head of hair throughout life (unless having a *neurogenic or desmogenic* sub-type*).

Neurogenic/Nervimotive
Comparisons *(Rocine)*

Attribute:	
Neurogenic	**Nervimotive**
Attitude	
patient, persistent, agreeable, calm	impatient, demanding, eager
Bust	
small	medium or large
Caution	
cautious	impulsive
Diet needed	
semi-vegetarian	carnivorous
Expression	
mild, kind	stern, critical
Fat	
little	may be a problem
Movements	
gentle, delicate	jerky, sudden
Voice	
sweet, loving	loud, persistent
Manners	
lovely, tasteful	persistent, firm
Nature	
feminine	masculine

Eyes — Blue or brown eyes with stiff and heavy eyelashes are the rule.

Ears —Your ears are of normal shape.

Nose —The nose is usually small or thin, some large and bony, and you may have a broad nose-tip.

Face — Your face is widest at the cheekbones, giving you a bony face (not fleshy) with vertical cheek lines.

▶ *The lower jaw is square at the angles of the jaw and often slopes down in a straight line towards the chin. The eldic and carbogenic types may also show a triangular face.*

Mouth and Lips —Your mouth may be drawn and set, the upper lip thin, the lower having variable shapes. Your voice is loud, commanding, authoritative, and matter-of-fact.

Teeth —Bright white teeth are the rule when healthy, or they may be yellow-white from mineral and trace-mineral deficiencies.

Skin —Thin and fine lines occur in the skin; color changes and freckles come and go with your mood and disposition.

Neck —The neck is muscular

Muscles — Your muscles are moderately strong; a unique coordination of mind, body, and speed may give you professional or Olympic athletic skills in tennis, football, basketball, baseball, swimming, etc. Great sports examples are Joe Montana, Joe Namath, John McEnroe, Jimmy Connors, James Worthy, Mark Spitz, and Sugar Ray Leonard.

Chest — The chest and lungs are strongly developed; the bust is usually moderate or large (most *neurogenic* and a few *nervimotive* types are small-busted).

Back and Shoulders — Your back and shoulders are broad, square, muscular, and strong.

Abdomen and Hips —The hips and abdomen are wide, flat, , and narrow from front to back.

Arms and Legs — The extremities are long, strong and bony. The palms are thick and often deeply lined.

Joints —The joints are strong and flexible

———

Nervimotive Personality Traits

If you are this Muscle type many, but not all, of the following characteristics are present—you may have overcome or moderated the negatives, but recognize that you once had several of them.

You may have any of these traits:

- Great business judgment
- Powerful willpower and passions
- Are very aggressive—never passive
- High sense of humor: many comics
- Willingly accept any disagreeable task
- Great workers with energy and tenacity

▶ *Rocine: "You have high intelligence with literary, artistic and intellectual talents: knowledge is craved, although you may not be so inclined while at school; when in the world you make up for lost time."*

- Are extremely industrious and hard working
- Sexual appetite is average, sometimes intense
- Brave and strong in battle, war, and emergencies
- High power of endurance (give 110% until exhausted)

- Usually highly motivated: concentrate and achieve any task
- Have executive and management ability (rarely liked as bosses)
- Have strong muscle and bone development; excel at sports; many professional sports figures
- Are very expressive with dislikes and complaints; have high self-confidence; inclined to depression, hopelessness, low self-worth

▶ *Rocine: "You are gifted conversationalists. You crave intelligent companionship on your own terms.... Many of you are attracted to learning, education, reputation, money, position, and power."*

Potential Challenges

▶ *If you relate to any of these challenges, doing something to overcome them serves your evolution.*

You may have evolved from or not experienced these general challenges, so do not dwell on this list. The negative aspects are potential traits that you may have evolved from, or not experienced.

► *Rocine: "Your faults are similar to those of the desmogenic. You are often impatient, intense, excitable, intolerant, impassioned, hot-tempered, and demand obedience."*

- Need to be in control
- High sense of gossip, litigation
- Tend to exact revenge for threats and wrongs
- Some may not be evolved, cultured or refined
- Combative, unpredictable, believe in "eye for an eye"
- Overly aggressive and pushy tendency; may easily make enemies
- Typically, you may desire or crave coffee, alcohol, pot, nicotine, and/or drugs
- Some have a dominating, sarcastic, and threatening attitude; may worry unnecessarily
- Attitude of "knowing it all" with a level of cockiness that unfortunately for your antagonists, you back up with deeds

———

Nervimotive Stress Management

You have poor mental stress prevention, causing you to internalize this stress into your stomach, adrenals, and immune system with disease potential. While living under stress conditions you need nerve nutrition like calcium/magnesium, and valerian root or chamomile herb, two capsules, twice daily with food. (You benefit by following the advice in Booklet #1. Your emotional stress prevention is not strong, and any of the above challenges may need reprogramming help. Do written releases of negative emotions as described in Booklet #2.)

———

Love

Romances are often fleeting unless you find your mate and love affinity, which is not easy. You have a high, even intense, ability to love but if unfulfilled in that love you may readily move on. Some of you become co-dependent in relationships. You are often attracted to the *carbogenic, neurogenic, pathoferic, nitropheric, and pargenic* types.

———

Talents and Vocations

Abilities —*Law, talk, teaching, literary, artistic, intellect, police, military, management, conversation, hard sales, show business, money making*

You have many attributes and talents. Your may waste your teen years because of parents not controlling your natural rebelliousness: you may drop out of high school, be a troubled child, or be easily tempted into alcohol or drug experimentation.

▶ *Rocine: "You should be successful because:*

- You have high executive and financial talents.
- Sulfur intensifies your emotions and passions.
- You have a keen perception of values and ethics.
- You have abilities in business, sales, and industry.
- You are able to study, learn, and apply life lessons.
- Calcium and phosphorus promote your brain metabolism."

▶ *I have known or observed you as singers, actors, accountants, comedians, psychologists, office managers, salesmen galore, football quarterbacks, and as professional athletes.*

Inabilities —*Science, healing, diplomacy*

You are not suited for painstaking scientific applications or the healing professions. The type information cannot predict what you will become, but you are capable of bringing a creative excellence or brilliance to whatever you do in life.

———

Health Problems

You are long-living, but tend to age early because of nervous intensity and nutritional exhaustion in your brain, bone and nerves.

▶ *Rocine: "Eating dairy foods and cooked sulfur foods is the root cause of your health problems; this results in intense passions, emotions, unhappiness, and impaired health."*

If sick, you commonly experience health problems or diseases in any of the following organs and tissues:

Retina — The retina is weak and vulnerable to mental stress.

Gastrointestinal Tract — Stress causes ulcers, colitis, etc.

Sexual Organs — Are predisposed to infections and female organ diseases, cysts, tumors, etc.

Nervous System —You are vulnerable to temper, insomnia, hair loss, nervous ailments, and head, neck and back pains (from mental stress).

Other — Chemicals, drugs, electrical fields, radiation, etc., affect you badly.

———

Nervimotive Acid/Alkaline Factor

For your health and healing, the genetics of your autonomic nervous system predispose you to needing a specific ratio of food acidity to alkalinity. You are born with an alkaline constitution, and predominantly need an **acid-ash** food intake for acid/alkaline balance. (Ash refers to the minerals left in your body after metabolizing a food.) Your autonomic nervous system genetics are *parasympathetic* dominant,

requiring about 70% proteins and carbohydrates, but…

> *For your healing, if in ill health or after about age 40-45, you need to aim for this approximate ratio of food selections:*
>
> > *50% Fruits, salads, vegetables*
> > *50% Proteins, carbohydrates*

[See Chapter 3 for details on this subject, along with the common symptoms found with people of different nervous system dominance.]

———

The Nervimotive Spiritual Factor

Skip this paragraph if uninterested in a philosophical perspective on your type!

▶ *Rocine: "The soul chooses the body type."*

If as souls, we choose the brain and body type to spend a lifetime in, it could be to learn certain spiritual lessons related to perfecting ourselves, and our humanity, in God's eyes. What lessons does the type bring you? Only you can really decide what those lessons are. You know your weaknesses, faults, and behaviors towards others. You know things about yourself that Victor Rocine could never get from his research subjects when he first wrote about types. So search your mind for the answers.

Each discrete type has challenges of life lessons, goals, etc., and some of yours may be:

Go-Go Nervous System — Your nervous system overloads with your thoughts, worries and stress, and is busy making ulcers!

Faith — Many of you have great faith.

Grudges — May hold grudges; give yourself permission to forgive others.

Controlling — You often demand obedience and control: if you want closer relationships meet people halfway (which may be difficult for you).

Aggression — Are dominating, may make enemies: calm down, therapy!

Imtience — Understand that others cannot do things as well as you can!

[Some of you accomplish all of these goals!]

———

A Nervimotive Story...

Leoni, age 29, 5'1, had jet-black hair, a shapely body, and a pleasant countenance. She was not diseased, but complained of constipation, palpitations, insomnia, nervousness, and fatigue. Examination showed a magnesium deficiency and I advised her to eat those foods daily. She also had mental stress overloading into her stomach and intestines, and key therapy was to nurture her nervous system (with calcium and B-complex). The dietary changes, implemented along with the herbs indicated for her type, resolved her symptoms within a few weeks.

Nervimotive Type Mineral Foods

*Apply this mineral data to the diet following
these Muscle type descriptions.*

Excessive Foods:

- *Calcium*
- *Carbon (simple carbohydrates)*
- *Sulfur (cooked)*
- *Sodium (salted, junk)*

Deficient Foods:

- *Phosphorus*
- *Magnesium*
- *Sulfur (raw)*
- *Sodium (unsalted, non-junk)*

*These deficient minerals are common deficiencies
in your type, and predispose you to ill-health. If ill,
be sure to use these lists with your <u>daily</u> food
intake. If not ill, eat from the foods lists 3-4 times
<u>weekly</u>. All food lists are in descending order of
concentration and value to you, choose servings of
foods in the upper half of each list first!
One serving is ½ cup (minimum).*

Nervimotive Excessive Foods -

Calcium is excessive in your tissues. It is highly concentrated in your bones, joints, muscles, nerves, heart, teeth, and gums, and if you have an illness or disease in any of these tissues, calcium excess may be a significant problem.

Carbon, excessive in all people who become fat or obese, is found in every cell of your body as the basis of all life.

Sulfur in *cooked* form is excessive in your tissues, such foods bringing excess sulfur acids into your tissues and emotional instability—raw sulfur foods preclude this happening.

Sodium from salted junk foods is excessive in your tissues. To preserve your health and weight control avoid junk foods and fulfill your sodium needs from the food list (without the salt shaker).

Deficient Foods –

In illness or disease, it is important to correct these mineral deficiencies.

Phosphorus is deficient in your tissues, and is needed because of intense nervous system activity and brain exhaustion from your thinking, planning, and worrying about health and everything in your life.

Magnesium is often deficient in your type, and is particularly important for your brain, heart, and digestive function.

Sulfur in raw foods is deficient (see above notes).

Sodium in food form, not as salted junk foods, is deficient (see above notes).

▶ *Approximate your food ratios. On any particular day, it does not matter if one meal is mostly alkaline and another mostly acid—just try to balance it out for the day! If you make a mistake, try again tomorrow. It is a subjective call that you make, and what is done over time that makes the difference to your health.*

———

<u>Minimize</u>
Excessive Mineral Foods

Calcium: *2-3 servings/<u>week</u>*

Swiss and cheddar cheese, turnip greens, almonds, brewer's yeast, corn tortillas, dandelion greens, brazil nuts, watercress, tofu, dried figs, sunflower seeds, yogurt, whole wheat, milk products, ripe olives, broccoli, cottage cheese, spinach.

Carbon: *1-2 serving/week*

Simple carbohydrates, fructose corn syrups, sweet fruits, whole grain cereals and breads, salt, all fast foods, packaged foods, canned and frozen foods, soy sauce, all preserved meats (cured, smoked, canned and luncheon meats), sauces (barbecue, catsup, etc.), dill pickles.

Sulfur (cooked): *0-1 serving/week*

Cabbage, onions, cauliflower, garlic, Brussels sprouts, broccoli, turnips, mustard greens, rutabagas, spinach, beans, carrots, horseradish.

[Avoid these acidic cooked foods: they are detrimental to your health: eat <u>raw</u> sulfur foods.]

And Minimize ...

Sodium (salted, junk): 0-1 *servings/week*

Salt, all fast foods, packaged foods, canned and frozen foods, preserve meats (cured, smoked, canned), sauces (soy, barbecue, catsup, etc.), chips (potato, corn, etc.), dill pickles, sauerkraut, bouillon cubes, peanut butter, salted nuts, crackers, or packaged soups, processed cheeses, commercial salad dressings, meat tenderizers.
Use the salt-shaker sparingly! Potassium salt is acceptable.

Note: If you must eat anything on the above list, keep it down to ½ cup weekly!

Note - The food recommendations are for the generic type. Additionally, you may need from a holistic healer or nutritionist something more specific for your individuality.

Eat
Deficient Mineral Foods

Phosphorus, Sodium (non-junk):
1-2 servings/day

Soda water*, seeds (pumpkin, kelp, sesame), scallops, squash, Swiss chard, beets and greens, celery, dried pinto beans, peanuts, egg white, cod, chicken, walnuts, cashews, rye, pecans, oats, carrots, parsley.
(* Not sugared soda <u>drinks</u>)

Magnesium: *1-2 servings/day*

Kelp, cashews, blackstrap molasses, buckwheat, dulse, filberts, peanuts, millet, pecan, walnuts, rye, beet greens, coconut, Swiss chard, collard leaves, shrimp, sweet corn, avocado, prunes (dried).

Sulfur (raw): *1-2 servings/day*

Cauliflower, cabbage, onions, garlic, spinach, horse-radish, carrots, radishes, almonds, chestnuts

Note: Eat any healthy foods you desire, but be sure to include the type foods in your daily choices.

Nervimotive Nutritional Supplements

- **Multi-Vitamins** *[Take all supplements with food]* —*2 capsules/day*

- **Magnesium**
  — 200 mg/day

- **Phosphorus**
  Obtain Phosfood tabs from a good Health Food Store (Standard Process Labs: take as directed on the product).

- **Do not take Calcium**
  You absorb it like a vacuum cleaner. (Exception: if highly stressed, menopause, on estrogen, osteoporotic)

- **Herbs**
  Brain detox —Vervain or Valerian Root
  Organ detox — Milk Thistle or Strawberry Leaf
  (Take one capsule, twice daily for one month; then one, three times weekly.)

- **Lecithin**
  —1,300 mg/three times weekly with food

- **Evening Primrose or Flaxseed Oil**
  —One soft-gel/day

Important Nervimotive Health Concerns

You stress yourself into diseases through excessive worrying, passions, excitement, and temper tantrums. You particularly need a brain and nerve diet high in magnesium and phosphorus (and low in cooked sulfur foods).

You often need affirmations to encourage positive thinking and to take command of your mental stress.

Your nervous system genetics require the *Muscle* type Food Guide for health, and any flesh cravings are normal and healthy for you. After about age 50, you need about four flesh days and three vegetarian days each week. Animal proteins should be limited to a few times weekly. You may choose to be vegetarian (not recommended), which requires you take a daily protein drink.

<u>*Nervimotive Food Guide*</u>

Aim for –

50% Proteins, complex carbohydrates
50% Fruits, salads, vegetables
and
70% Cooked foods
30% Raw foods

Avoid salt!
Avoid dairy foods and cooked sulfur vegetables!
Accomplish mental balance!
Take the recommended supplements.

Nervimotive Weight Loss

Losing weight depends upon you following the type instructions, summarized in this section. The males seldom have weight problems; reducing calorie intake readily addresses them. For females, their weight loss is more complicated because of several factors, in particular:

- *Stop* eating carbon foods
- *Eat* body type deficient mineral foods daily
- *Follow* your *Nervimotive* food guide food instructions

- *Exercise*: your body type requires moderate daily exercise
- *Simple sugars*: stop all white table sugar and high-fructose corn syrup and drinks containing these sugars
- *Mental balance and positive thinking:* you are very easily mentally stressed by everyday life, which causes adrenal hypoglycemia, low blood sugar; you need to take these supplements: *calcium/magnesium*, two capsules, twice daily with food; and *chamomile*, two capsules with food
- *Hypoglycemia:* this hormonal imbalance stops fat loss, and usually initiates more fat production, so it is vital to deal with this problem: take *pantothenic acid*, 500 mg/twice daily with food (see my earlier books to resolve this problem)
- *Calories:* As with any dietary approach, calories in, must be *less than* calories out! Most markets sell a calorie booklet; make notes of your daily intake, and in most instances keep it under about 1500 calories/day
- If the above fails to help you, be sure to refer to my earlier books for help with your hormones and liver function.

———

Muscle Types
General Food Guide
(Carnivores)

Important Note

———

The Food Guide addresses the <u>Acid-Alkaline</u> aspect of your food intake, along with the <u>Type Mineral</u> factor presented throughout this book. It does <u>not</u> necessarily address calories or other dietary factors that may be pertinent to your personal health needs whether medical or appropriate for some other dietary need. So use your common sense and just include the factors described here with whatever healthy dietary choices you usually make.

For other nutrient information, consult with nutritional books or with holistic nutritional doctors. I particularly recommend the advice of Andrew Weil, M.D.

———

Muscle Types
General Food Guide

(Not for the Nitropheric Type)

This chapter presents a general Food Guide, upon which you superimpose the nutritional information from your type chapter. As a Muscle body type your genetics require flesh foods.

Meat/Flesh Intake

Most muscle types should limit red meat to once or less weekly, while eggs, lamb, fish, or poultry are excellent in moderation. If ill or diseased, be sure to eat daily, one or two servings from each *deficient minerals* list. If not ill, eat them at least three times weekly for health maintenance. If this diet is similar to your present diet, but healing is sluggish, then:

- Decrease your carbohydrate and protein intake by about one-third
- Increase your fruit, salad, and vegetable intake by about one-third
- Consult with a holistic doctor, preferably one versed in nutritional and emotional evaluation

---

Over-Acid or Over-Alkaline?

Just as a log of wood burned in your fireplace leaves a mineral-ash, food ash refers to the minerals remaining after metabolizing foods in your tissues:

- Fruits, vegetables **alkalinize** tissues
- Proteins, carbohydrates **acidify** tissues

Usually You Are Over-Acid Due To:

- Excessive intake of dairy foods
- Excessive intake of proteins and carbohydrates
- Deficient intake of fruits, salads and vegetables
- Accumulated metabolic waste-acids (from years of eating excessive acid-ash foods, meats and carbohydrates, and from lack of exercise)
- You need to estimate the ratio of foods eaten. Generally, eat the following *approximate* ratios for your health:

> 50% <u>**Alkaline-ash**</u> foods *(fruits, salads, vegetables)*
> 50% <u>**Acid-ash**</u> foods *(complex carbohydrates like starches, grains, cereals, breads, flour products; and proteins)*

Approximate your food ratios. On any particular day, it does not matter if one meal is mostly alkaline, and another mostly acid—just try to balance it out for the day! If you get it wrong, try again tomorrow. It is a subjective call that you make, and it is what you do over weeks, months, or years that make the difference—not on any one or two days.

Note - If Vegetarian

As a general indication, if you follow a vegetarian diet substitute vegetable sources of protein for the any flesh in the food guide. Note that contrary to most alkaline-ash vegetarian diets you need something different:

*You need an **acid-ash** vegetarian diet high in complex carbohydrates and vegetable proteins.*

Because of your high need for protein, you usually require a vegetable powdered protein supplement in juice (about 25-30 grams daily).

Important

- Minimize white sugar and alcohol intake.
- If desired, interchange lunches for dinners.

- Never eat foods you are allergic to, no matter what I recommend; if allergic, or suspect a food allergy, eliminate it and substitute from your type mineral lists.
- Eat the right foods 80-90% of the time and the Food Guide will work for you; unlike some types you do not have to live out of a health food store (although such foods are healthier for you).

▶ *Omit eating the excessive minerals in your type chapter, and be sure to eat one or two servings from the deficient list daily.*

Finally, in addition to your body type needs, other holistic healing matters also need your attention. I strongly suggest that you refer to my web site and earlier books for that information: *DrStenbeck.net*

———

Acid/Alkaline Genetics Chart

The following chart reflects each Muscle Type and its acid or alkaline-ash food needs. These ratios change if you are unhealthy or over age 45-50. Refer back to your body type and review the *Acid/alkaline* instructions.

———

Dr. Lloyd Stenbeck

Acid/Alkaline Genetics, Dietary-Ash, and Raw Food Needs

This chart shows the Rocine types, their acid or alkaline food needs, and the percentage of raw foods needed for your health and healing.

- Apply the Type Minerals to the Food Guide -

Type	Acid/Alkaline Genetics	% Food-Ash Needed	% Raw Food Needed
Calciferic	Alkaline	70% acid	30
Carbogenic	Alkaline	50-50	50
Desmogenic	Alkaline	70% acid	50
Eldic	Intermediate	50-50	50
Medeic	Intermediate	50-50	50
Myogenic	Intermediate	50-50	50
Nervimotive	Alkaline	70% acid	50
Nitropheric	Acid	70% alkaline	70
Pallinomic	Alkaline	50-59	30

The above percentages vary depending on aging and the health of individual types.

Muscle Types / Food Guide
<u>Breakfast</u>

[Superimpose the nutritional information from your

EGGS* (1-2) with lettuce, tomato, or salad, whole grain toast; (add bacon or sausage 1-3 times weekly if desired)
— 2-4 times/week; or

FRUIT fresh salad, and protein (yogurt, milk, cheeses, seeds, nuts)
—1-3 times/week; or

CEREALS, with fruit, seeds, nuts
—2-5 times/week; or

OTHER choices
— 0-1 times weekly

<u>Daily liquids:</u>
Pure water, citrus, vegetable juices, soups, other —as desired
Coffee, teas —0-2 cups

[Include selections from your type mineral needs everyday.]

Muscle Types / Food Guide

Lunch

SALADS, *mixed green, protein (poultry, fish, egg, cheese, seeds or nuts, etc.), whole grain breads*
[Dressing: olive oil/vinegar; low-fat, low-cal dressings]
— 2-4 times/week; or

SANDWICH, whole grains with a protein (cheese, tuna, ham, etc.); and salad and/or vegetables
— 1-4 times/week; or

POULTRY OR FISH, 3-6 oz., with a mixed green salad and/or vegetables
—1-3 times/week; or

OTHER choices (with salad or vegetables)
—1-2 times/week

[Other oils permitted, but less ideal is soybean oil, a common allergen; minimize commercial dressings. Be sure to include two or more selections from your type food lists in your daily food intake. For in-between meal snacks, eat fruit or vegetables with seeds/nuts.]

Muscle Types / Food Guide
Dinner

POULTRY OR FISH *(4-6 oz.), with salad and/or vegetables*
—2-4 times/week; or

PASTA *with protein (chicken, etc.) with salad and/or vegetables*
— 2-4 times/week; or

VEGETARIAN *meal with salad and/or vegetables*
—1-3 times/week; or

LEAN BEEF *(4-6 oz.) with salad and/or vegetables*
— 0-1 times/week

OTHER *choices with salad and/or vegetables*
— 0-1 times/week

Desserts:
Fruits, fresh —as desired
Low-sugar, healthy desserts
— 0-3 times/wk

Dr.Lloyd Stenbeck

Food Guide Notes

Steamed Vegetables —

Minerals are lost in the boiling of vegetables; steaming or wok cooking is best.

Food Combinations —

If you have a weak digestive system then eating proteins at the same meal with starches often results in indigestion, gas, or constipation.

Periodic Detox —

You tend to over-indulge in acid-ash foods (proteins and carbohydrates), and often need occasional elimination diets for tissue waste-acid removal. Have a holistic doctor or nutritionist supervise such detox (where you have an alkaline-ash diet along with protein supplementation).

Minimize —

- Fatty foods
- Commercial salad dressings
- Beef, red meats, processed meats
- Coffee, white sugar, corn syrup, alcohol

Vegetarian Proteins —

You require a carnivorous diet. An exception is the *nitropheric* type who functions best with a *vegetarian* diet. The other muscle types are born to be carnivores. It is very difficult for the other muscle types to be pure vegetarians because of their strong intuitive cravings for fish, poultry, meat, or eggs. If you are vegetarian, then because of your high needs for amino acids and acid-ash foods, you should take a protein supplement of 30-40 grams/day (powdered protein in juice).

Healthy Weight —

Several of you gain weight as the ravages of age, lack of exercise and dietary excesses take their toll. By eating according to your body type, you should naturally lose excess weight. Each type also has a few individual factors that only apply to them!

You have a good ability to lose weight by following the Food Guide instructions. The most common problem I find with your weight-control is liver and kidney irritation due to food allergies, which results in extra pounds. The key is to eat non-allergic foods.

If drinking more than 3-4 cups daily of coffee or tea, you may have a hypoglycemic problem (low blood sugar), which contributes to making fat, ill-health, and delayed healing. (Refer to the earlier books for help with this healing.)

———

Appendix

Brief Extracts from
<u>The 22 Unique Body Types</u>

———

Appendix A

Types
(Brief extract)

Type comes from 'typus' meaning an image or impression, the study of types being called typology.

▶ *Rocine: "A combination of mental and structural features is consistently found in people of the same type."*

Rocine wrote that all types are a mixture of positive and negative qualities. He based his work on the biochemical individuality of our *mineral* absorption and utilization. Of course, all minerals are absorbed, but he postulated that different types of people *selectively* absorb certain minerals, to a greater or lesser extent, requiring specific mineral foods for their enhanced health and healing. This is the basis of his types.

▶ *The type information cannot predict what or who you will become, or how successful or not, but your type is capable of bringing a creative excellence to whatever you do in life. If your type has negative qualities that you disagree with, remember that they are only tendencies and may or may not manifest in you.*

This book enlarges on Rocine's premise (early 1900's), integrated with the later research of Herbert Sheldon, M.D., Ph.D., at Harvard University (1930's), along with my fifty years of observations and experience with this subject.

Comparing your shared physical (and sometimes psychological) descriptions with the Celebrity Lists further assists the identification of your type. It is not that you will look exactly like, or be a twin to, any particular celebrity. Look closely at a celebrity's features: face, profile, height, weight, head, etc. If you know something about their talents, beliefs, success and failure spheres, health and weight challenges, attitudes and behaviors, etc., then you get clues as to what your type may be.

———

Understanding Types and Sub-Types

Each of us has a clearly discernible dominant type. Visualize the celebrity examples from movies, politics, sports, the arts and public life, and try to identify with their physical features. Look for similar features, remembering that you will not recognize all attributes in yourself. You are not looking for your twin!

The sub-type issue is the main reason people of the same major type can look so different. Remember that a type description does not characterize you exactly, but depicts your individual variant of a type.

▶ *The type questionnaire pinpoints the major features of that type: if the celebrity examples are unhelpful, you may be an unusual variant (in which case ignore the celebrity issue and give yourself 7 points on Question 1).*

———

Minerals

Minerals are essential life nutrients that accelerate enzyme and chemical reactions and provide a basis for your body typing. Although found in all tissues, different minerals tend to be concentrated in certain organs, their presence or absence contributing to the healing of such tissues; e.g., zinc accelerates prostate healing; calcium and manganese promote bone, joint and connective tissue healing.

Specific foods nurture each type, some people needing meats for their health others needing a vegetarian diet. A high potassium diet nurtures one person, while another needs high sulfur, calcium, zinc, or another mineral.

Mineral Digestion and Absorption

Compared to vitamins, minerals are *difficult* to digest, absorb, and utilize. In people with strong digestive systems, this aspect may not be important. The following factors should be in place for optimal mineral metabolism:

1. Stomach Hydrochloric Acid Production
2. Parathyroid Hormone Balance
3. Organ Toxic Metal and Chemical Removal
   [See details in The 22 Unique Body Types.]

─────

Total Body Healing

Note that from a holistic healing perspective, in addition to minerals and type information, attend to these healing factors:

> *Nutrient Balance*
> *Mental Balance*
> *Emotional Balance*
> *Spiritual Balance*
> *Detoxifying Integrity*

The above factors are all important to your total healing especially if you are interested in self-healing (see my earlier books).

———

Researchers
(Brief extract)

The predominant workers in this area of human individuality from around 1880's to the 1960's are Herbert Sheldon, M.D., Ph.D., Roger Williams, Ph.D., and Victor Rocine, D.Sc.

Much information on Sheldon's research exists on-line and in medical psychology libraries; for interested readers there is other research published in the last century. This book is primarily about Rocine's body types.

Herbert Sheldon M.D., Ph.D.

In contrast to Rocine, Sheldon at Harvard University in the 1930's was trained in the scientific method and did painstaking research and publishing on human individuality. In comparing his findings with Rocine's work, a direct putative correlation is visible.

Roger J. Williams, Ph.D.

Another significant researcher in human individuality is the renowned scientist and biochemist, Roger J. Williams. He demonstrated that different people have varying levels of nutrients, enzymes, and other metabolic chemicals in their bloodstreams.

▶ *Williams's research firmly expands on the premise of individual nutritional needs in human beings. If interested in his research, I highly recommend his book <u>Biochemial Individuality</u>.*

Victor Rocine, D.Sc.

Note that when a negative feature is indicated, say neurotic tendencies, all members of the type are <u>not</u> that way; it is a type tendency reported by Rocine.

Rocine studied type-related diseases finding links between mineral and dietary factors with individual types and their diseases. In each body type, one or more dominant minerals are preferentially absorbed and utilized over other minerals.

He recognized discrete body types from their physical appearance finding genetically based mineral dominance to be the determining feature. He also correlated their physical features with psychological characteristics.

———

Genetics, Types, and Diet
(Brief extract)

This section deals with how nervous system genetics helps determine your eating choices for health: you are either born to be a predominant meat eater, a partial or complete vegetarian, or something between the two. The genetic factor determining this dietary aspect is the *sympathetic and parasympathetic* components of your central nervous system. This represents a basic factor in eating for health.

This chapter helps you understand your dietary inheritance, although instinctively, you may already have arrived there!

- If born **sympathetic** dominant you are *genetically acid*, desiring a predominantly *vegetarian* diet for your health (about 70% fruit, salad, vegetables to 30% proteins and carbohydrates).

- If born **parasympathetic** dominant you are *genetically alkaline*, desiring a predominantly *carnivorous* diet for your health (70% proteins, carbohydrates). Few of you ever choose to become vegetarian because of the difficulty in satisfying your protein needs.

- If born ***intermediate*** dominant you may eat food groups with little concern for the acid/alkaline factor. However, after age 40, you need a semi-vegetarian diet for healthy eating.

———

Chart of Relative Nervous System Dominance

In the following Chart, if you relate to many of the symptoms on one side you probably have that nervous system dominance; relating to both sides indicates *Intermediate* dominance.

If Vegetarian (Over-acid)
>*Eat 70% fruits, salads, vegetables*
>*And 30% proteins, carbohydrates*

If Carnivore (Over-alkaline)
>*Eat 70% proteins, carbohydrates*
>*And 30% fruits, salads, vegetables*

If Intermediate
>*Eat 50:50 of acid and alkaline-ash foods*

Make an *approximate* estimate of your daily acid and alkaline food intake (such ratios varying from type to type).

———

Symptoms of Relative
Genetic Dominance

Vegetarians (Over-acid)	Carnivores (Over-alkaline)
Sympathetic Dominance	*Parasympathetic Dominance*
little or no flesh desire	desire flesh
easily constipated	rarely constipated
slow digestion	fast digestion
easily dehydrated	not dehydrated
strong thirst	low thirst
pale face	flushed face
high pulse after food	slow pulse after food
easy gag reflex	slow gag reflex
cool dry skin	moist warm skin
nervous stomach	calm stomach
little eyelid blinking	much blinking
nervous tendency	mostly calm
slower healing	faster healing
low oxygen-uptake	good oxygen-uptake
easily breathless	seldom breathless
insomnia common	sleep easier
few muscle cramps	some night cramps
calcium deposits rare	get calcium deposits

Appendix D

Help Identifying your Body Type with Dr. Stenbeck

If you desire help in identifying your body type, follow these instructions, and answer the questionnaire. For further information and fees, send me an email from page one of the website:

DrStenbeck.net

First name: _____

Country of birth: _____

Upload photos and send to the above website:

- Head and shoulders: front and side views
- Full body: front and side views
- Also 1-2 teenage views
- If possible, casual photos of mother, father, siblings

MY TYPE CLASS MAY BE: _____

  (Thin, Muscle, or Fat)

AGE   -   _____

HEIGHT   -   _____ feet/inches

MY WEIGHT -   __ _____ pounds

- Heaviest at age: _____

- Lightest as adult: _____

- Estimate age 15: _____

VISION - Excellent   Average   Poor:

HAIR - Natural color: _____

 - Thin/thick? _____

 - balding? _____

SKIN - Quality: _____

   - History of acne, boils, other:

_____

_____

TEETH -   Strong   Weak   Dentures

 - Cavity history: Many   Moderate   Few

MUSCLES   -   Strong   Average   Weak

      Sports played _____

JOINTS -   Strong   Average   Weak

HEALTH - Childhood diseases?

_____

_____

 - Adult diseases?

_____

AVERAGE DIET

- Beef _____ (times/week)

- Poultry _____ (times/week)

- Fish _____ (times/week)

- Eggs _____ (times/week)

- Water _____ (glasses/day):

- Vegetarian? Vegan? _____

- Other? _____

- Did your childhood diet differ? _____

The above will help me know who you are! I will send you a follow-up questionnaire for further help in identifying your body type.

Appendix E

On-line Health Consultation with Dr. Stenbeck

For further information, or to comment on this book, or to receive a response on any health issue from a holistic viewpoint, send an email inquiry from page one of my website:

DrStenbeck.net

Following that, I will suggest further healing needs, which we may pursue with an on-line consult.

———

Appendix F

Notes

See my book *The 22 Unique Body Types*, available at the usual online source, for further information and details on all of the 22 Types. The Appendix in that book also has more information about:

- *Mineral Functions and Food Sources*

- *Further Reading*

———

www.ingramcontent.com/pod-product-compliance
Lightning Source LLC
Chambersburg PA
CBHW062101280526
45788CB00003B/1299